45 Effective Juice Recipes to Naturally Control Your High Blood Pressure:

45 Home Remedy Solutions to Your Hypertension Problems

By

Joe Correa CSN

COPYRIGHT

ACKNOWLEDGEMENTS

This book is dedicated to my friends and family that have had mild or serious illnesses so that you may find a solution and make the necessary changes in your life.

45 Effective Juice Recipes to Naturally Control Your High Blood Pressure:

45 Home Remedy Solutions to Your Hypertension Problems

By

Joe Correa CSN

CONTENTS

ABOUT THE AUTHOR

After years of Research, I honestly believe in the positive effects that proper nutrition can have over the body and mind. My knowledge and experience has helped me live healthier throughout the years and which I have shared with family and friends. The more you know about eating and drinking healthier, the sooner you will want to change your life and eating habits.

Nutrition is a key part in the process of being healthy and living longer so get started today. The first step is the most important and the most significant.

INTRODUCTION

45 Effective Juice Recipes to Naturally Control Your High Blood Pressure: 45 Home Remedy Solutions to Your Hypertension Problems

By Joe Correa CSN

These recipes will help you to quickly and naturally lower your blood pressure in a matter of hours. High blood pressure is a serious health condition we all have to face sooner or later. Some people have the tendency to develop it earlier and others (the majority) once they pass the age of 50. High blood pressure is not something we have to be afraid of, we just have to learn how to control it, the sooner the better. It is for these reasons that we have prepared a selection of powerful juice recipes. Keep in mind how valuable your body is and that we should not wait until this condition gets worse. Prevention is the key!

We have included juice with fruit combinations with strawberries, blueberries, lemons, and many more because of the high vitamin C concentration in them and their powerful effect's on dilating blood vessels. We also included juices with watermelon, linseed, bananas, and others because of their high levels of potassium which is an essential element when trying to control hypertension. Some juice recipes have celery and parsley for their phytochemicals and their capacity to eliminate toxins from your body and help control high blood pressure levels.

Make sure to take high blood pressure seriously and make a conscious decision to lower it by controlling what you eat on a daily basis.

45 EFFECTIVE JUICE RECIPES TO NATURALLY CONTROL YOUR HIGH BLOOD PRESSURE: 45 HOME REMEDY SOLUTIONS TO YOUR HYPERTENSION PROBLEMS

1.   Banana power (4 people)

Ingredients:

- 2 bananas cut in slices
- 2 cups of orange juice
- 4 spoons of natural honey
- 4 spoons of linseed powder
- 8 ice cubes
- 4 eggs
- 1 spoon of lemon juice

Procedure: In the blender mix the banana with the orange juice for 30 seconds. Add the sugar, linseed powder, ice cubes and mix again for 50 more seconds. Add the egg and mix for 5 seconds. Serve in 2 large glasses and pour the lemon juice on top.

Nutritional facts: Energy 298 kcal, total fat 0 g, cholesterol 0 mg, carbohydrates 26 g and fiber 5 g.

2.   Avocado and mango juice (2 people)

Ingredients:

- 1 cup of mango cut in slices

- 1/2 cup of avocado cut in cubes

- 2 spoons of honey

- 1/2 cup of natural yogurt

- 1/2 cup of green tea

Procedure: Put the fruits into the fridge for 10 minutes. Mix everything in a blender until you get a creamy look. Add water progressively if you want a more liquid mixture. Serve immediately.

Nutritional facts: Energy 243 kcal, total fat 3 g, cholesterol 7 mg, carbohydrates 69 g and fiber 10 g.

3.   Aloe vera and papaya juice (2 people)

Ingredients:

- 1 aloe vera leaf
- 1 cup of papaya cut in cubes
- 2 spoons of honey
- 1/2 cup of water
- 1/2 cup of ice cubes

Procedure: Cut the base, lower part and peak of the aloe vera leaf. Let rest in water what is left for 48 hours. Then open cutting the skin in the middle and with a spoon take all what's inside. We will call this alove vera pulp. In a blender mix the papaya, a cuarter of cup of the aloe vera pulp, honey as you like, water and ice.

Nutritional facts: Energy 142 kcal, total fat 0 g, cholesterol 0 mg, carbohydrates 34 g and fiber 2 g.

4.   Camu Camu shake (6 people)

Ingredients:

- 3 spoons of camu camu powder or 1 cup of camu camu cut in cubes
- 1 cup of water
- 2 cups of papaya cut in cubes
- 2 cups of strawberries
- 1/2 cup of ice in cubes
- 2 spoons of natural honey

Procedure: In a blender mix the camu camu, strawberries and the ice. Add the honey and mix. Serve in 4 glasses. You can join this powerful shake with oat pancakes

Nutritional facts: Energy 100 kcal, total fat 0 g, cholesterol 0 mg, carbohydrates 22 g and fiber 3 g.

5.   Fenugreek smoothie (2 people)

Ingredients:

- 1/4 cup of fenugreek seeds powder
- 1 cup of papaya cut in cubes
- 1/2 cup of green tee
- 1/2 cup of lactose free milk
- 2 spoons of sesame seeds
- 2 spoons of honey

Procedure: Mix everything in a blender until you get a creamy look. Add water progressively if you want a more liquid mixture. Serve in large glasses.

Nutritional facts: Energy 245 kcal, total fat 0 g, cholesterol 0 mg, carbohydrates 46 g and fiber 8 g.

6. Tropicalmelon shake (4 people)

Ingredients:

- 3 cups of papaya cut in cubes
- 1 cup of mango cut in cubes
- 1 cup of watermelon cut in cubes
- 2 cups of natural yogurt
- 1 ½ cups of pineapple cut in cubes
- 1 cup of ice cubes
- 2 spoons of linseed powder

Procedure: In a blender mix all the ingredients until you get a creamy look. In case you may need something to dissolve if the juice is too dense you can use half cup of water. Serve in long glasses.

Nutritional facts: Energy 194 kcal, total fat 4 g, cholesterol 7 mg, carbohydrates 35 g and fiber 5 g.

7.   Non-toxins juice (4 people)

Ingredients:

- 6 strawberries cut in cubes
- 4 chopped plums
- 2 almonds
- juice from ½ lemon
- 2 spoons of raw beetroot
- 2 spoons of grated carrots
- 1 apple cut in cubes without skin
- 1 cup of green tee

Procedure: In a blender mix all the ingredients until you get a creamy look. In case you may need something to dissolve if the juice is too dense you can use half cup of water. Serve in long glasses.

Nutritional facts: Energy 162 kcal, total fat 3 g, cholesterol 8 mg, carbohydrates 64 g and fiber 2 g.

8.   Mango and coconut (3 people)

Ingredients:

- 2 cups of coconut juice
- 1 ½ cup of mango cut in cubes

Procedure: You can get coconut juice by cutting a coconut on the top until you break the shell. In case you have no access to fresh coconut you can also use coconut essence by mixing 20 ml of it with 2 cups of water. In a blender mix the coconut juice and the mango. Avoid using honey because the mango has its own natural sweetener. Serve in 2 tall glasses.

Nutritional facts: Energy 149 kcal, total fat 1 g, cholesterol 0 mg, carbohydrates 35 g and fiber 3 g.

9. Strawberry and orange shake (4 people)

Ingredients:

- 1 cup of natural yogurt
- 1 banana
- 1 cup of orange juice
- 8 strawberries

Procedure: Take the green part out from the strawberries and wash. In a blender mix all the ingredients until you get a creamy look. Serve in long glasses.

Nutritional facts: Energy 213 kcal, total fat 0 g, cholesterol 0 mg, carbohydrates 38 g and fiber 3 g.

10. Mint shake (3 people)

Ingredients:

- 1/2 banana
- 1/2 cup of strawberries
- 1/2 cup of orange juice
- 2 mints leafs
- 1 cup of green tee

Procedure: In a blender mix all the ingredients until you get a creamy look. In case you may need something to dissolve if the juice is too dense you can use half cup of water. Serve in long glasses.

Nutritional facts: Energy 232 kcal, total fat 10 g, cholesterol 19 mg, carbohydrates 46 g and fiber 4 g.

11.   Peach shake (4 people)

Ingredients:

- 2 cups of peach cut in cubes
- 1 cup of natural yogurt
- 1/3 cup of pineapple cut in cubes
- 1/4 cup of water

Procedure: In a blender mix all the ingredients until you get a creamy look. In case you may need something to dissolve if the juice is too dense you can use half cup of water. Serve in long glasses.

Nutritional facts: Energy 206 kcal, total fat 11 g, cholesterol 6 mg, carbohydrates 54 g and fiber 7 g.

12.   Fenugreek fantasy (2 people)

Ingredients:

- 2 cups of fenugreek juice

- 1 cup of chopped parsley leafs

- 2 spoons of sesame seeds

- 1 spoon of linseed powder

- 2 spoons of honey

Procedure: The fenugreek juice is the water from boiling the seeds. You should boil 4 cup of seeds in ½ liter of water in order to get the juice. Then mix everything in a blender until you get a creamy look. Add water progressively if you want a more liquid mixture. Serve in large glasses.

Nutritional facts: Energy 222 kcal, total fat 0 g, cholesterol 0 mg, carbohydrates 48 g and fiber 6 g.

13.   Coconut - lemon (5 people)

Ingredients:

- 3/4 cup of lemon juice

- 4 spoons of natural honey

- 1 cup of coconut cream

- 6 ice cubes

- 1/2 cup of coconut in slices

- 1 grated lemon

Procedure: In a blender mix 1 liter of water, lemon juice, honey, coconut cream and ice. Serve and decorate with the coconut and the grated lemon.

Nutritional facts: Energy 234 kcal, total fat 9 g, cholesterol 16 mg, carbohydrates 54 g and fiber 4 g.

14.   Delicious Mango (4 people)

Ingredients:

- 2 cups of watermelon cut in slices
- 2 bananas cut in slice
- 1 mango cut in cubes
- 1 cup of natural yogurt
- 1 spoons of natural honey
- 1 cup of ice cubes

Procedure: In a blender mix the watermelon, bananas and mango. Add gradually the yogurt until you get a creamy look. In case you may need something to dissolve if the juice is too dense you can use half cup of water. Add the ice cubes and mix again. Serve in long glasses.

Nutritional facts: Energy 256 kcal, total fat 4 g, cholesterol 8 mg, carbohydrates 68 g and fiber 4 g.

15.   Almonds shake (2 people)

Ingredients:

- 1 cup of natural yogurt

- 1 spoon of peanuts (without salt)

- 2 spoons of toasted oats

- 1 spoon of toasted sesame seeds

- 1 spoon of almonds

- 2 spoon of natural honey

Procedure: In a blender pour the glass of almonds milk; add the wheat germ, oats, sesame and almonds. Dress with honey. Serve immediately.

Nutritional facts: Energy 259 kcal, total fat 9 g, cholesterol 14 mg, carbohydrates 32 g and fiber 7 g.

16.   Cranberry juice (1 people)

Ingredients:

- 1 cup of organic cranberry juice (250 ml)
- 1/2 cup of water
- 1 spoon of olive oil
- 2 spoons of natural honey

Procedure: Take all the ingredients to the blender and mix until you get a creamy look. It's recommendable to take it every day before breakfast.

Nutritional facts: Energy 198 kcal, total fat 1 g, cholesterol 1 mg, carbohydrates 43 g and fiber 4 g.

17.   Watermelon juice (2 people)

Ingredients:

- 4 cups of fresh watermelon
- 3 spoons of fresh parsley leafs
- 1 spoon of natural honey

Procedure: Chop the parsley leafs. Put the watermelon in the blender and mix until you have a liquid and fluid look. Add honey to dress. Serve in tall glasses and pour the basil on top.

Nutritional facts: Energy 187 kcal, total fat 0 g, cholesterol 0 mg, carbohydrates 46 g and fiber 5 g.

18.   Parsley juice (2 people)

Ingredients:

- 1 cup of fresh parsley
- 1 green apple
- juice of ½ lemon
- 1/2 spoon of grated ginger
- 1 cup of water

Procedure: Chop the parsley and apple. Introduce all the ingredients to the blender and mix. Strain the juice. Serve in large glasses. Drink before breakfast

Nutritional facts: Energy 222 kcal, total fat 4 g, cholesterol 0 mg, carbohydrates 57 g and fiber 5 g.

19.   Lemon juice (2 people)

Ingredients:

- 8 lemons

- 2 glasses of water

- 2 spoons of apple vinegar (30 ml)

Procedure: Squeeze the juice from the lemons and mix with the water and vinegar. To clean your body and kidneys take the juice during mornings at least during a week.

Nutritional facts: Energy 159 kcal, total fat 0 g, cholesterol 0 mg, carbohydrates 32 g and fiber 2 g.

20.   Fenugreek milkshake (2 people)

Ingredients:

- 1 cup of fenugreek juice

- 1 cup of almond lactose free milk

- 1/4 cup of chopped almonds

- 2 raisins cut in slices

- 2 spoons of honey

Procedure: Mix everything in a blender until you get a creamy look. Add water progressively if you want a more liquid mixture. Serve in large glasses.

Nutritional facts: Energy 228 kcal, total fat 9 g, cholesterol 28 mg, carbohydrates 46 g and fiber 7 g.

21.   Celery and apple juice (2 people)

Ingredients:

- 2 celery steam including the leafs
- 3 apples
- 1 spoon of fresh mint
- 2 spoons of honey
- 1/2 cup of water

Procedure: Cut the celery, apples and mint. Put everything in a blender and mix until you get a creamy look. If you want it more liquid then you should add water progressively until you get the look you are looking for. Strain the juice and serve.

Nutritional facts: Energy 215 kcal, total fat 0 g, cholesterol 0 mg, carbohydrates 58 g and fiber 3 g.

22.   Carrots and celery juice (1 people)

Ingredients:

- 3 big carrots

- 3 celery steams

- 1 cup of water

Procedure: Wash the carrots and the celery. Peel the carrots and then cut in slices. Chop the celery. Put the ingredients in the blender and mix. Serve in tall glasses.

Nutritional facts: Energy 154 kcal, total fat 0 g, cholesterol 0 mg, carbohydrates 27 g and fiber 4 g.

23.   Cucumber and parsley juice (2 people)

Ingredients:

- 1/2 cucumber

- 100 gr of parsley

- 1 cup of water

Procedure: Wash the cucumber and parsley. Cut the cucumber in slices and chop the parsley. Put everything in the blender and mix. Strain and serve.

Nutritional facts: Energy 176 kcal, total fat 0 g, cholesterol 0 mg, carbohydrates 35 g and fiber 2 g.

24. Grape juice (2 people)

Ingredients:

- 250 g of red grapes
- 1 cup of water
- 1/2 spoon of mint
- 2 spoons of honey

Procedure: Wash the grapes. Peel the grapes and then cut by the half to take the seeds out. Put everything in a blender and mix. Serve immediately.

Nutritional facts: Energy 165 kcal, total fat 0 g, cholesterol 0 mg, carbohydrates 36 g and fiber 4 g.

25.   Watermelon and lemon juice (2 people)

Ingredients:

- 4 cups of fresh watermelon cut in cubes
- 4 spoons of lemon juice
- 1/2 cup of water
- 2 spoons of honey

Procedure: Mix everything in a blender until you get a creamy look. Dress with honey and mix again. Serve in tall glasses.

Nutritional facts: Energy 175 kcal, total fat 0 g, cholesterol 0 mg, carbohydrates 28 g and fiber 3 g.

26.   Watermelon and celery juice (2 people)

Ingredients:

- 3 cups of watermelon

- 3 celery steams

- 2 spoons of natural honey

- 1 cup of water

Procedure: Wash the celery. Peel the watermelon and cut in thin slices. Chop the celery. Join together with the water in a blender and mix. Strain and serve in tall glasses.

Nutritional facts: Energy 176 kcal, total fat 0 g, cholesterol 0 mg, carbohydrates 31 g and fiber 2 g.

27.   Body cleaner juice (2 people)

Ingredients:

- 1/2 cabbage
- 1 carrot
- 2 celery steams
- 1/2 cup of germinated beans
- 1 cup of pineapple
- 1 cup of water

Procedure: Mix everything in a blender and add water progressively. Once you have a creamy look you are ready to strain the juice. Serve and enjoy.

Nutritional facts: Energy 232 kcal, total fat 2 g, cholesterol 2 mg, carbohydrates 47 g and fiber 6 g.

28. Acai-berry mix juice (2 people)

Ingredients:

- 1/2 cup of orange juice
- 1 banana cut in slices
- 1 mango cut in slices
- 1 cup of pulp of acai berries
- 1 cup of water
- 2 spoons of natural honey

Procedure: Mix everything in a blender and add water progressively according to the consistence you want to get. Once you have a creamy look serve and enjoy.

Nutritional facts: Energy 276 kcal, total fat 10 g, cholesterol 9 mg, carbohydrates 64 g and fiber 5 g.

29. Blood pressure special juice (2 people)

Ingredients:

- 4 carrots
- 2 apples
- 1 piece of ginger (5 cm)
- 1/2 cup of coconut juice
- 1 cup of water

Procedure: Wash all the ingredients. Peel the carrots and ginger. Chop the carrots and apples. Mix everything in a blender. Serve immediately.

Nutritional facts: Energy 245 kcal, total fat 4 g, cholesterol 7 mg, carbohydrates 43 g and fiber 4 g.

30.   Fenugreek and papaya juice (2 people)

Ingredients:

- 1 cup of fenugreek juice

- 1 cup of papaya cut in cubes

- 1 cup of green tee

- 2 spoons of sesame seeds

- 2 spoons of honey

Procedure: Consider that the fenugreek juice is obtained by boiling the seeds in a pot with ½ liter of water. The water you get from it is the juice, you can reserve the rest for the next days and mix it with your juices. Now mix everything in a blender until you get a creamy look. Add water progressively if you want a more liquid mixture. Serve immediately.

Nutritional facts: Energy 245 kcal, total fat 3 g, cholesterol 8 mg, carbohydrates 76 g and fiber 8 g.

31.　Pumpkin juice (2 people)

Ingredients:

- 1 glass of water
- 1 glass of coconut juice
- 1/2 cup of cooked pumpkin
- 1 spoon of honey

Procedure: In a blender mix the coconut, water and pumpkin for some minutes until you get a creamy look. Pour the juice in tall glasses and add the honey and mix again. Enjoy.

Nutritional facts: Energy 198 kcal, total fat 2 g, cholesterol 6 mg, carbohydrates 66 g and fiber 4 g.

32. Blueberry juice (2 people)

Ingredients:

- 1 cup of natural yogurt
- 1 cup of blueberries
- 1 spoon of linseed powder
- 1/4 cup of water

Procedure: Wash the blueberries. Mix everything in a blender until you get a creamy look. Add water progressively if you want a more liquid mixture. Serve immediately.

Nutritional facts: Energy 198 kcal, total fat 11 g, cholesterol 21 mg, carbohydrates 54 g and fiber 2 g.

33. Orange shake (2 people)

Ingredients:

- 1 cup of orange juice
- 1/2 cup of water
- 1/2 spoon of vanilla essence
- 2 spoons of honey
- 1/2 cup of natural yogurt
- -5 ice cubes

Procedure: Mix everything in a blender until you get a creamy look. Add water progressively if you want a more liquid mixture. Serve immediately.

Nutritional facts: Energy 212 kcal, total fat 3 g, cholesterol 6 mg, carbohydrates 48 g and fiber 2 g.

34.   Apple-carrot juice(2 people)

Ingredients:

- 2 cups of orange juice

- 1 cut of chop apple

- 6 carrots cut in cubes

- 2 spoons of honey

Procedure: Mix everything in a blender until you get a creamy look. Add water progressively if you want a more liquid mixture. Serve immediately.

Nutritional facts: Energy 198 kcal, total fat 5 g, cholesterol 2 mg, carbohydrates 62 g and fiber 5 g.

35.   Super banana booster (2 people)

Ingredients:

- -3/4 cup of milk

- 1/4 cup of granola

- 1 banana

- 1 cup of ice cubes

- 2 spoons of linseed powder

Procedure: Mix everything in a blender until you get a creamy look. Add water progressively if you want a more liquid mixture. Serve in tall glasses.

Nutritional facts: Energy 276 kcal, total fat 7 g, cholesterol 7 mg, carbohydrates 32 g and fiber 7 g.

36.   Spinach banana (2 people)

Ingredients:

- 1 banana

- 1/2 cup of chopped spinach

- 1 spoon of peanut butter

- 1 ½ cup of lactose free milk

- 1 spoon of linseed powder

- 1 spoon of sesame seeds

Procedure: Mix everything in a blender until you get a creamy look. Add water progressively if you want a more liquid mixture. Serve in tall glasses. Decorate with sesame seeds and enjoy.

Nutritional facts: Energy 230 kcal, total fat 9 g, cholesterol 9 mg, carbohydrates 23 g and fiber 7 g.

37.   Kale power juice (2 people)

Ingredients:

- 1 cup of fresh kale

- 1 cup of almond milk

- 1 cup of blueberries

- 1/2 banana

- 1 spoon of almond butter

- 2 spoon of instant oats

Procedure: Mix everything in a blender until you get a creamy look. Add water progressively if you want a more liquid mixture. Serve immediately.

Nutritional facts: Energy 256 kcal, total fat 9 g, cholesterol 8 mg, carbohydrates 25 g and fiber 12 g.

38. Blueberry-oats juice (2 people)

Ingredients:

- 1 banana
- 1 cup of blueberries
- 1/3 cup of instant oats
- 1 cup of lactose free milk

Procedure: Put the banana and blueberries in the fridge for 10 minutes. Mix everything in a blender until you get a creamy look. Add water progressively if you want a more liquid mixture. Serve in tall glasses.

Nutritional facts: Energy 214 kcal, total fat 4 g, cholesterol 0 mg, carbohydrates 64 g and fiber 4 g.

39.   Red delights (2 people)

Ingredients:

- 1/2 cup of raspberries

- 1 cup of strawberries

- 1 cup of mango

- 1 cup of water

- 2 spoons of honey

Procedure: Put the fruits into the fridge for 10 minutes. Mix everything in a blender until you get a creamy look. Add water progressively if you want a more liquid mixture. Serve immediately.

Nutritional facts: Energy 214 kcal, total fat 5 g, cholesterol 0 mg, carbohydrates 48 g and fiber 4 g.

40.   Blue delights (2 people)

Ingredients:

- 1 cup of raspberries

- 1 cup of blueberries

- 1 cup of strawberries

- 1/2 cup of natural yogurt

- 1/2 cup of green tee

Procedure: Mix everything in a blender until you get a creamy look. Add the water progressively if you want a more liquid mixture. Serve in tall glasses.

Nutritional facts: Energy 198 kcal, total fat 4 g, cholesterol 5 mg, carbohydrates 38 g and fiber 4 g.

41.   Straw-nana juice(2 people)

Ingredients:

- 1/2 cup of chopped pineapple

- 1 banana

- 1/2 cup of mango cut in slices

- 1 cup of strawberries

- 1 cup of lactose free milk

Procedure: Mix everything in a blender until you get a creamy look. Add water progressively if you want a more liquid mixture. Serve immediately.

Nutritional facts: Energy 215 kcal, total fat 3 g, cholesterol 6 mg, carbohydrates 53 g and fiber 5 g.

42.   Green delights (2 people)

Ingredients:

- 1 chopped kiwi
- 1 ½ cups of watermelon cut in cubes
- 1 ½ cups of red grapes
- 1 cup of lactose free milk
- 1 spoon of vanilla essence
- 1 spoon of honey

Procedure: Peel the grapes and then cut by the half. Take all the seeds out and chop. Mix everything in a blender until you get a creamy look. Add water progressively if you want a more liquid mixture. Serve immediately.

Nutritional facts: Energy 245 kcal, total fat 6 g, cholesterol 7 mg, carbohydrates 48 g and fiber 5 g.

43.   Mango delights (2 people)

Ingredients:

- 2 mangos cut in slices

- 1 cup of natural yogurt

- 1 cup of water

- 1 banana

- 2 spoons of lemon juice

- 1 spoon of vanilla essence

Procedure: Mix everything in a blender until you get a creamy look. Add water progressively if you want a more liquid mixture. Serve in large glasses.

Nutritional facts: Energy 198 kcal, total fat 3 g, cholesterol 7 mg, carbohydrates 46 g and fiber 4 g.

44. Apple and lemon juice(2 people)

Ingredients:

- 2 green apples cut in cubes

- 6 leafs of kale

- 2 steams of celery

- 1/2 spoon of lemon juice

- 1 cucumber

Procedure: Wash and chop the kale, cucumber and celery. Mix everything in a blender until you get a creamy look. Add water progressively if you want a more liquid mixture. Serve in large glasses.

Nutritional facts: Energy 187 kcal, total fat 3 g, cholesterol 0 mg, carbohydrates 56 g and fiber 4 g.

45.   Raspberry-mint delight (2 people)

Ingredients:

- 2 cups of raspberries cut in cubes
- 1 cup of water
- 3/4 of natural yogurt
- 1 cup of chopped mango
- 1/2 cup of chopped mint leafs
- 1 spoon of lemon juice
- 1 pinch of salt
- 1/2 cup of ice cubes

Procedure: Take the fruits to the fridge for 10 minutes. Mix everything in a blender until you get a creamy look. Add water progressively if you want a more liquid mixture. Serve immediately.

Nutritional facts: Energy 243 kcal, total fat 3 g, cholesterol 7 mg, carbohydrates 54 g and fiber 7 g.

ADDITIONAL TITLES FROM THIS AUTHOR

70 Effective Meal Recipes to Prevent and Solve Being Overweight: Burn Fat Fast by Using Proper Dieting and Smart Nutrition

By

Joe Correa CSN

48 Acne Solving Meal Recipes: The Fast and Natural Path to Fixing Your Acne Problems in Less Than 10 Days!

By

Joe Correa CSN

41 Alzheimer's Preventing Meal Recipes: Reduce or Eliminate Your Alzheimer's Condition in 30 Days or Less!

By

Joe Correa CSN

70 Effective Breast Cancer Meal Recipes: Prevent and Fight Breast Cancer with Smart Nutrition and Powerful Foods

By

Joe Correa CSN